Celia Johnson has had a varied life. Unable to choose between being a professional musician and a nurse, she initially combined the two careers. While travelling the world on orchestral tours, she would give her colleagues first aid, massage and reflexology. Her enthusiasm for preventive and complementary therapies eventually took over and she gave up playing to focus on building her massage practice. She became a full-time therapist in 1989.

She was so concerned about the problems experienced by therapists that she set up a support group. New therapists often asked her for advice, so that the idea of writing a book began to germinate, the result being *How to be a Successful Therapist*. As well as a busy practice, she also lectures to nurses on complementary therapies, runs workshops on setting up in business and has had several papers published in professional journals. She is married, has two daughters and lives in Guildford, Surrey.

HOW TO BE A SUCCESSFUL THERAPIST

Celia Johnson

Illustrations by Emma Dodd

The Book Guild Ltd
Sussex, England

First published in Great Britain in 2003 by
The Book Guild Ltd
25 High Street
Lewes, East Sussex
BN7 2LU

Typesetting in Times by
Keyboard Services, Luton, Bedfordshire

Printed in Great Britain by
Athenaeum Press Ltd, Gateshead

A catalogue record for this book is
available from the British Library

ISBN 1 85776 624 5

*To my clients and colleagues, from whom
I have gained so much*

CONTENTS

FOREWORD BY CLARE
MAXWELL-HUDSON

I was delighted to be asked to write the introduction to this new book on *How to be a Successful Therapist* not only because Celia Johnson has been known to me for years as a fellow professional, but also because I think that the ground she covers is of vital importance to the modern complementary therapist.

The concepts and ideas in this book have come from Celia's own personal experience. And personal experience leads to an understanding of the real requirements of building a practice, especially in a field such as this one. She has covered every aspect of becoming a successful therapist in a comprehensive yet humorous way.

I only wish her book had been available to me when I first set out in this field.

It is the capacity to care which gives life its deepest significance.

Pablo Casals

Your training is complete. Your certificates hang on the wall. You are a fully-fledged complementary therapist. Where do you go from here?

This book is intended to help you decide what you want from your complementary therapy business and how to go about achieving it. I have written it in response to the many enquiries I receive about setting up in practice. I hope it helps you to develop a satisfying and productive business.

For convenience I have grouped information in sections, but there is much overlap in topics. Although the book is intended mainly for massage therapists, it would also be of interest to other newly qualified complementary and beauty therapists.

1

SETTING GOALS

No wind blows in favour of a ship that has no port of destination.

Montaigne

What sort of a person are you? Are you single, married, divorced? Do you live alone, share with friends or live with your family? Are you planning to work in a big city, a small town, or a tiny village? Is the area affluent or poor? All these factors will influence the kind of practice you could set up.

What sort of practice do you envisage? You might choose to work:

- from home
- in a complementary therapy clinic
- doing home visits or on-site massage
- in a GP's surgery
- in a physiotherapy, osteopathic, or chiropractic clinic
- in a leisure centre
- at a health farm
- at a hairdresser's or beauty therapist's
- at a combination of the above

You might offer:

- a clinical environment
- a homely atmosphere

1

- incense and New Age music
- your front room, with the children watching TV and the dog barking!!!!!!

Finding your niche

Much will depend on your background and past career(s). In order to be successful you will need to find your niche in the market. Ask yourself why people would prefer to see you rather than therapist B down the road. What makes your treatment special? Are you good at de-stressing people? Are you good at remedial work? Are you a good listener?

I have a nursing background. I receive a lot of referrals from physiotherapists, doctors and osteopaths. I have a basic knowledge of how the body works (and what happens when it doesn't!). I treat lots of bad backs, arthritis and the like, and I know my limitations in practice. I also lecture to nurses on massage and complementary therapies.

A colleague (who isn't a nurse) is just as busy as I am, concentrating on de-stressing businessmen. We are both established in massage. We are successful because we have thought about what we are good at and have worked to develop that as an area of practice.

This is extremely important. There are many people training in complementary therapies, and standards vary enormously. You will need to sell not only your therapy, but your ability as a therapist and your personality as well. It may take time to develop confidence in yourself as a therapist, but if you are competent, professional in your attitude, and welcoming, people will come to see you. If you make them feel that you really care about them and that they are important to you, they will keep coming back!

2

SETTING YOUR WORK PATTERN

Where there is no vision the people perish.
The Book of Proverbs

Working hours

Planning the hours you will work may not seem terribly relevant when you see only a couple of clients per week. However, you expect your practice to grow, and it is important that it grows in a way *you* want, that it doesn't take you unawares. It is frustrating to find that you have scheduled only one client every day, when they could have been scheduled one after the other on just one or two days a week, allowing you to use your time more fruitfully. It is important to treat people when it is convenient for both you and the client, so that you are not constantly at their beck and call just because you need the money! If you do that, you will become exhausted and less efficient as well.

You need to consider these questions:

- How many hours/days per week do you plan to work?
- How many treatments will you do per day?
- Will you offer evenings and weekends?
- If so, how many and how late?

Where to work

Work is love made visible.
Kahlil Gibran, The Prophet

It is perfectly possible to earn your living working in a variety of places. If you wanted, you could, for example, do one day a week in a clinic, one day at a health farm, two days at home and one day making home visits. Such variety can be good, because you have all the advantages of each workplace without getting too bogged down with the disadvantages. You will have to choose what works best for you. The following reflects the choices available.

Complementary therapy clinics

There are now clinics in most cities, towns and villages in the UK. Some charge a sessional rate plus deposit, while others ask a percentage of your takings. The percentage rate can work to your advantage when you are starting out and may not have many clients.

Points to consider about a clinic:

- Will you get on well with the owner?
- Will you be allowed to work in the way you choose?
- How many other therapists in your discipline also work there?
- Who are the other therapists and what are they like?
- Where is the clinic situated?
- Are there adequate parking facilities for you and your clients (and does it matter if there are not)?
- Is the equipment provided, such as the couch, suitable for you?
- What other support will be provided? Will you have access to receptionists, telephone, fax, photocopying,

washing facilities, towels, or couch covers?
- Will the clinic provide any clients or do you have to find them all yourself?
- Are there likely to be any additional costs, such as advertising?
- Who 'owns' clients in the event that you move on from the clinic?
- How much notice do you have to give when leaving?
- What flexibility is there over the hours your room is available?
- Under what circumstances would you lose your deposit?

Working in a clinic which is a local centre of excellence can be a great start for the fledgling therapist. The clinic will already be attracting the right clientele and you will gain a lot from the stimulation of being with other, more experienced therapists. There are likely to be people around when you need advice. You do not lose privacy as you would when working at home, and most equipment will be provided for you.

This sounds ideal and it can be. But let's look further. Are you sure that this really *is* a thriving clinic, or is it just a building where 30 therapists come for half a day each and fight for what little work there is? Assure yourself that the person who uses the room before you leaves it in a habitable state. Look carefully at the owner. I once worked in a clinic where the owner insisted on seeing all new clients herself for a first consultation. The theory was that she would then refer to other therapists as appropriate. In fact she continued to treat them all herself, while telling us that we were not making enough effort to attract clients!

In another clinic, the owner insisted that all therapists be trained in an additional discipline, as she wanted all

5

clients to be treated in a particular way. She charged the therapists a lot of money for her training, and they had very little say in the way they could work.

Having said all that, I have kept in touch with many of the therapists that I met while working in clinics. They were all extremely good at their job and I have learned a great deal from them.

The advantages of working in a clinic:

- It is a suitable environment and equipment is provided.
- You have a ready-made address and phone number.
- Cleaning and heating are provided.
- Photocopying and fax facilities are usually available.
- It may be a ready-made source of clients.
- You may gain support and stimulation from other therapists.
- It is likely to be advertised locally and should attract appropriate clientele.
- You suffer no loss of privacy and no wear and tear on your home.

The disadvantages of working in a clinic are:

- It will involve some financial outlay, regardless of income.
- There may be competition from other therapists.
- The owner may expect you to fit in with his or her views about treatment.
- Rent increases are beyond your control.
- The owner may try to take the larger share of clients.
- Clients may not be allocated fairly among therapists.
- You may not be allocated sufficient time for each treatment.

Working at home

Your house is your larger body.
Kahlil Gibran, *The Prophet*

There are a significant number of therapists who work at home. This is often the simplest option when starting out, as it involves the least financial commitment.

Points to consider about working from home:

- Do you have a suitable room to use for treatment?
- Do you need planning consent or a licence from your local council?
- Can you provide a quiet environment?
- Can you heat just that room without affecting your entire home?

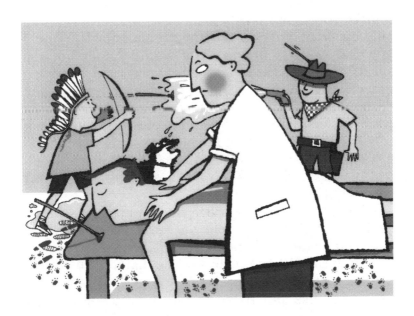

- How will you cope with the additional laundry?
- Do you have parking facilities (and does it matter if you do not?)
- Do you mind having strangers in your home?
- Do you mind people making personal comments about your home, decor and/or garden?

Working at home may seem ideal, but it is actually a mixed blessing. There is no extra outlay for rent, but loss of privacy is a big disadvantage. You may feel that this is not a problem when you see only a couple of people per week. But once your practice grows, it becomes more of an issue, when you could have 20 or more people tramping through your home.

It is also more difficult to exercise control over who comes to your home, particularly if you advertise. Spend time talking to people when they phone – not only does it make you seem friendly and interested, but it is also a vital opportunity to sift out anyone undesirable. Should you end up with anyone you would rather not see again, you can be left feeling rather vulnerable. However, it has been my experience that unsuitable clients usually do not return, or even make appointments in the first place – those requiring the services of a prostitute do not continue to waste time on the phone to a massage therapist! (One man even told me that maybe he would like a real massage one day – no doubt after his visit to the prostitute!)

Whether or not you choose to work from home depends on the suitability of your living accommodation, whether you can provide parking, and how quiet the environment is. However much you plan for this, family and friends may have other ideas.

A psychotherapist friend tells of seeing a new client for the first time on the day her 18-year-old left school.

The girl had celebrated in the pub with her friends and returned home incapable of coordinating key and lock. She rang the doorbell endlessly, while the poor psychotherapist tried to concentrate on her client. As she ushered him out, her drunken daughter fell through the door. The client was still within earshot as the psychotherapist yelled furiously at her daughter! (The client continued to see her for four years, so it wasn't a total disaster!)

It is worth mentioning that not all clients like 'whale music' and incense. Do bear in mind that some people really treasure silence and their preferences should be respected.

Another possible disadvantage of working from home is that you will need to buy all your own equipment, such as a couch and towels. I would suggest that you buy as good quality a couch as possible. You are likely to spend a lot of hours working at it, so it is worth taking time and trouble to find one that is right for you. If you have the space, consider a hydraulic or electric couch. They are not as expensive as you might think and will give you much greater flexibility as you work.

I buy my towels from a local market stall. They are 'seconds' but perfectly good and much cheaper than from a shop. You will also have to wash them or use a laundry service. My washing machine takes enough towels for two clients. If you do six treatments a day, your washing machine will have to take three loads of towels before you have done any personal laundry. Laundry services are worth looking into. There are some which can provide the towels as well as washing them. They can also help if your washing machine lets you down. My local dry cleaner also does a service wash which I use in a crisis.

You should contact your local council to find out

whether or not you need a licence to work from home and whether you need planning consent. It's better to write than to phone the council, as you want to have their reply in writing. That way, if a problem should arise, you've got something more concrete than vague assurances that some nameless person on the other end of the phone told you!

It is usually necessary to obtain planning consent only if the room is used *exclusively* for work. If you use your treatment room for work 8 hours a day and for the remaining 16 hours it is a library/study/spare bedroom, you should not need planning consent.

The advantages of working at home:

- The work environment is within your control (in theory anyway!).
- You have complete autonomy over the way you work.
- There is no financial outlay for rent/deposit.
- It is easier to absorb fluctuations in income.
- If you have young children, you may still be able to work if they are unwell.
- Your clients may prefer it.

The disadvantages of working at home:

- You may feel isolated.
- You may appear less professional than if you were working away from home.
- There may be no one around if you are treating someone you're unhappy with.
- You have to buy all the necessary equipment yourself.
- You pay the cost of heating, lighting and laundry.
- You pay the cost of advertising.
- The onus is on you to find clients.
- You have loss of privacy.

- Noises of children, doorbells, the telephone or TV may cause distraction.
- Clients may phone at inconvenient times because they know you are there.

Home visits

Where you are there arises a place.

Rilke

Home visits are worth considering if your own home is not suitable and you do not wish to work in a clinic.
Questions to consider about home visits:

- Do you have a car to transport the couch?
- Is your 'portable' couch truly portable?
- Do you have an answering machine/mobile phone?
- How much will you charge for travelling time?
- How large an area are you prepared to cover?
- Are you good at map reading?
- Can you work comfortably on someone else's 'home ground'?
- Are you good at finding a suitable spot to work in someone else's home?
- Are you good at keeping to schedule?
- Are you easily waylaid by offers of cups of tea or clients who are not ready when you arrive?
- Are you able to adapt what you do to fit the client's environment?
- Do you like animals? Some clients regard their pets as part of the family and may insist they stay with you during the treatment.
- You will need to allow extra time for setting up.

Remember to take into account the time you will spend

11

travelling and the wear and tear on your car (and on you, carting your couch around). It may be that the room you do the treatment in is up lots of flights of stairs. It could be barely big enough to get your couch into, making it difficult to work properly. You won't know any of this until you have been somewhere for the first time. You will also need to be aware of the need for extra vigilance in someone else's home. A colleague tells of the time she went to do some waxing. The client's young son burst into the room and knocked over the pot of hot wax onto the new, immaculate (until then) carpet! I once caught an antique vase with my bag and knocked it onto the floor. Fortunately it didn't break. On another occasion I had to treat a client with a large Labrador sitting on my feet. It refused to move until I had given it some massage!

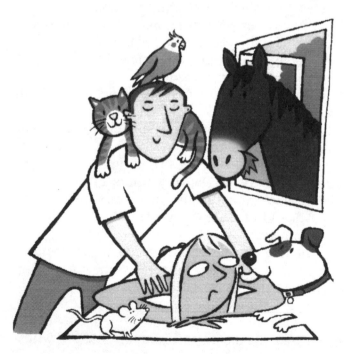

The advantages of home visits:

- You suffer no loss of privacy.
- There is no wear and tear on your furniture and carpets.
- You have no substantial financial outlay, assuming you already have a car.
- The client bears the cost of heating and lighting.
- Clients can relax afterwards instead of having to get themselves home.

The disadvantages of home visits:

- They may not provide an ideal work environment.
- You may not be easy to contact if away from home for long periods.
- You suffer wear and tear on your car.
- It is more difficult to impose a time schedule in someone else's home.
- Great care is needed to avoid spills or breakages.

Health farms

Health farms are often looking for complementary therapists, and if you like the idea it is worth contacting any near you. You will probably earn more per treatment working elsewhere, but you will gain lots of experience which is useful when you are setting out. It also looks good on your CV or brochure to say that you have worked there. A disadvantage is that you will not see clients long term, but you will certainly grow in confidence as you deal with such variety.

Doctors' surgeries

At the time of writing, NHS funding is in a state of flux.

In the past, GPs have been able to refer their patients to complementary therapists and the Primary Care Group paid the therapist. GPs remain responsible for the patient's care, so they will need to reassure themselves that you, the therapist, are competent. They may also prefer you to have some experience. Offering them a free treatment is a good way of introducing yourself. Be prepared to show some evidence of training, such as certificates and your CV.

Osteopaths/chiropractors/physiotherapists

They may have a room you could rent on a sessional basis and, being in complementary practice themselves, are more likely to identify patients you could help. You would need to be interested in and knowledgeable about bodywork and be able to work with other health professionals. They might expect you to have some experience and would probably appreciate seeing your certificates and CV.

Hospices/homes for the elderly/hospitals

The way to get in to these areas is often to offer to work voluntarily, but it is possible that you could be paid. Some therapists begin as volunteers and progress to being paid at a later date.

Do not be downcast if your offers are rejected. Keep offering your services and you will find your niche. I repeat that it is important to know what you want and aim for that. Don't waste time chasing job opportunities which you know are not suitable for you.

3

MAKING A NAME FOR YOURSELF

Advertising

The gods only go with you if you put yourself in their path.

Aristotle

What to avoid

Unfortunately, people will read into your advert what they choose to see, which is not necessarily what you have written. All general advertising carries the risk that it will attract nuisance calls (see later chapter). You therefore have to be extremely careful how you word your advert to avoid any misunderstanding. Words such as 'service', 'caring', 'personal', 'friendly', 'mature', 'enjoy', and even 'Swedish', are often misconstrued. At all costs I would avoid using the word 'relief' in an advert, even if it is preceded by 'stress'. Further, any reference to personal appearance is not relevant to anyone seeking genuine massage.

Words conveying a professional image include 'treatment', 'alleviate', 'clinical', 'therapy', 'qualified', 'appointment' and 'therapist'.

Where to advertise

Newsagent or Post Office   An inexpensive way to advertise is to place a postcard at your local newsagent's

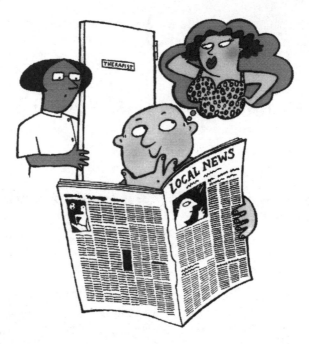

or Post Office. As long as it is worded carefully, it can bring you valuable local clients.

Local paper   If you pay for an advertisement in your local paper, particularly if you take one on a regular basis, the editors may be prepared to give you editorial space. You will normally be expected to write your own article, but remember that the newspaper will edit, particularly the last paragraph. Newspapers are keen to attract regular advertisers and may offer you discounts or special rates. There is no harm in asking, anyway. For some reason boxed adverts attract fewer nuisance calls, so it is worth bearing this in mind. My local paper agreed to instigate a new advertising column, 'Natural Therapies', when a group of therapists asked for it.

Yellow Pages and Thomson Guide   Although these

advertisements are comparatively expensive, they can be a reasonable source of new clients. You should advertise in the 'Complementary' or 'Alternative Health' section. The directory staff are themselves aware of the problems associated with advertising massage and will do their best to help you produce a professional advert. They also offer a choice of payment options so you don't have to find all the money in one go.

Targeting a particular market

Think about the kind of clients you would like to treat. Where would they be likely to hear about you? Approach health clubs, swimming and leisure centres, golf clubs and anywhere else you can think of. If they don't have a vacancy for you to work there, ask to leave your brochures *and keep returning to top them up.* Be sure always to have copies of your brochure and/or business card with you. (I keep some in my handbag and in the glove compartment of the car.) You could also ask to leave them with:

- local chemists
- hairdressers
- dentists
- doctors' surgeries
- physiotherapy clinics
- osteopaths/chiropractors
- chiropodists
- libraries
- health food shops (NB – many are only willing to take a business card due to lack of space)
- New Age bookshops
- Citizens' Advice Bureaux
- Environmental Health Departments at local councils
- Tourist Information

Self promotion

The Internet

When first starting out in practice, a website is unlikely to be a high priority, but as you gain experience in practice, or open a clinic, you might like to consider setting up your own site. It is impossible to vet who is looking at your site, so for your own safety you should speak to clients by telephone before agreeing to treat them. Many clients prefer a personal recommendation in any case. They are therefore more likely to ask a friend, rather than look for a therapist on the internet.

Remember that not all the information you find on the internet is accurate. You will need to be cautious about what you find, although there are, of course, genuine therapists and organisations who have their own sites. Some of these are listed at the end of the book. For example, *Positive Health* magazine runs an excellent website. It allows you to read articles from the magazine as well as link up with related topics on the world-wide web.

The most effective form of advertising or marketing is that which you undertake yourself.

Free treatment vouchers

Life takes it out of you. Massage puts it back.
Clare Maxwell-Hudson

It is worth offering vouchers for treatment to local charities to raffle or auction. If the voucher is not taken up, you have lost nothing. If someone comes for a treatment you will give your time, but they will probably come back if they enjoy it, and will tell their friends about you. Your name will also be mentioned at the time of the raffle, which is good advertising for you.

Talks to groups

You cannot teach a man anything. You can only help him discover it within himself.

Galileo

Giving talks to groups such as National Childbirth Trust, Women's Institute, charities, luncheon clubs and the like is also an excellent way of getting your name known. In my experience, the more talks you give, the easier it becomes. It is good to keep reaffirming your belief in your therapy and you may well gain new clients. You are unlikely to be paid much for giving talks, but you should be able to cover your expenses. (I ask for the cost of petrol and babysitting.)

Radio talks

It's no big trick to play the piano when you're *not* nervous.

Rudolph Serkin, pianist

It is unlikely that you will be offered the chance to speak on the radio early in your career. However, it is worth calling the radio station if you have a particularly interesting idea. If you are offered an interview, it is likely to be at very short notice – often the same day. It is therefore worth having a 'skeleton' talk or some questions and answers prepared in case you are asked to give a talk or interview right away.

As an alternative to your local radio station, a nearby hospital may have its own radio station. They may want you to give a talk in which you promote your own field of therapy but, in my opinion, it would be inappropriate to advertise yourself directly, unless invited to do so by the radio presenter.

19

It is natural to feel nervous about giving radio talks, but usually interviewers will be encouraging, and do their best to put you at ease. The most daunting interview I gave was alone in a studio with my microphone, while the interviewer was a hundred miles away in another studio! Watch out for leading or trick questions and keep as closely as possible to your prepared talk.

Take a blank tape with you so that you can have a recording of your talk. It is useful to know how often you said 'er' and how you could improve on your talk another time.

Making contacts

It isn't just knowing you can do something, it's allowing it to happen.

Wendy, riding instructor

Making contacts can be a very daunting prospect for most newly qualified therapists. However, there are things you can do to begin getting your business off the ground.

Networking

Make sure all your friends and work colleagues know what you do. Even if they don't come to you themselves, they may recommend you to others. Offer them some brochures to hand out to people they know. Word of mouth is the best way of attracting clients, but it does take time. Don't forget to keep in touch with your training school. Some keep a register of therapists from which to give names to enquirers. I have also gained clients from these sources:

- neighbours
- my children's school (parents and staff)
- the stables where I ride
- the postman (who sent a colleague with a bad back)
- taxi drivers

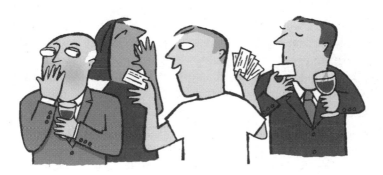

Other health professionals

You could try sending a letter to physiotherapists, doctors, dentists, osteopaths, chiropractors and chiropodists. Follow it up with a phone call to see if they would like any more information. You may like to offer them a free treatment so they can experience the benefits first-hand. It is good to develop a link with a practice, as they may 'sell' you to their clients. A referral from another professional is more valuable than any amount of advertising.

You could also phone other therapists in your discipline (the phone book and local paper should provide these). Make friends with them and assure them that you don't want to tread on anyone's toes. Established therapists can be a helpful source of advice and may pass on work when they are able.

Contact other complementary therapists too. Your local homeopath, herbalist, acupuncturist, psychotherapist, naturopath, and reflexologist may all be delighted to hear from you. They can also help you maintain your own health.

I once organised a therapists' supper. About eight therapists from different disciplines came for a meal. Each brought a dish to share, and their business cards. We had such a good evening that we decided to make it a regular event. Now, not only are we all able to refer clients to one another, but we all gain enormously from the stimulation of discussion and mutual support.

Sending formal letters to other health professionals is discussed in a later chapter. They are also a means of establishing contact and reputation with these individuals in the first place. I wrote to a GP after treating a lady I was unable to help. When another patient asked the doctor if he could recommend a massage therapist, he looked up my letter in the first lady's notes and referred the new patient to me.

Personalised literature

First, a word about spelling. What you practise in your practice is complementary therapy. You will have much greater credibility if you can spell what you do!

Brochures

The first point to consider is what you intend to use your brochures for. Possibilities include:

- mass marketing – putting them through local letter boxes, under car windscreens, etc.
- targeted marketing – placing them in a variety of appropriate outlets.
- personal marketing – handing them out personally at health exhibitions.

Your brochure or leaflet is your opportunity to tell the world about your therapy and yourself. It should persuade all those reading it that they should come to see *you*. It should be a true reflection of you and your practice (or what you intend your practice to be). Most of us progress through several leaflets or brochures, reflecting the changes as our practice grows and develops. I felt at a loss when designing my first brochure, but soon began to enjoy writing about my great passion – massage. If you are enthusiastic about your therapy, others will pick up on that and they will want to know more.

Your brochure should be written with potential clients in mind. What would they want to know that would persuade them to come and see you? Broadly, I would suggest that brochures should contain the following kinds of information:

- your therapy – what it is, its benefits and who might benefit from it
- the therapist(s) – a brief professional background, including your qualifications and anything which distinguishes you from the competition
- a phone number (no need to give your address)

Your brochure may also show:

- a photograph of you and/or your treatment room
- testimonials from satisfied clients
- your hours of work
- details of your fees
- approximate length of consultation
- your policy on charging for cancellations
- a convenient time to phone you

Get someone you know to read your draft and give constructive comments before finalising the text. *You* may think that it is wonderful but a good friend can always improve it!

Having decided on the content, you will have to choose how you will produce your brochure. The advent of desktop publishing and the home computer may enable you to produce something yourself, though you may well find that using your own desktop facilities for print runs of over 1000 can be expensive and time-consuming. It may be better to use a local photocopying facility or a quality printer. The choice will probably be determined by whether you choose to include a photograph or graphics and the quality of the paper or card that you wish to use for your brochure.

Some pitfalls to avoid in brochures include:

- spelling mistakes
- poor grammar
- giving too much information which discourages the reader
- an imbalance between the amount of information on the therapy and on the therapist
- poor quality paper/colour/print
- too much information on potential side effects/reactions of the therapy

Business cards

Business cards are cheaper than brochures to produce and are useful when you make personal contact with potential customers. They are less likely to be effective if they are left for people to pick up. If you have spoken to a person about your therapy and its potential benefits, a business card is a useful reminder of who you are. It may also be passed on by someone who is recommending you to a friend.

Business cards should give:

- your name
- qualifications
- types of therapy
- a telephone number (no need to give an address)
- email/website if you have them

They are easy to keep in a wallet, pocket or handbag, and may also double as an appointment card.

Headed notepaper, compliment slips and treatment vouchers

In order to appear professional in your dealings, you will need to have headed notepaper, compliment slips and vouchers (if you plan to use them). You may like all your personalised literature to match, but this is not essential. Your stationery should be good quality, reflecting the fact that you are offering a quality service.

Curriculum vitae

Preparing a CV is a useful discipline whether you are setting up your own practice or seeking employment. It can help you identify where your individual advantage might lie, for it is this which distinguishes you in the eyes of your client or prospective employer. Although I am self-employed, I have also been asked for a summary of my professional life by doctors before they would consent to refer patients to me.

Many people embarking on careers in complementary therapies have come from a completely unrelated background or have just completed their full-time education. If this is true for you, how do you show that you are competent when this field is all new to you?

In fact, if you look back over your life to date, you may well find something which links your past and present careers. Perhaps you have had experience in dealing with certain groups of people, such as the elderly or the young, and this connection can be presented as an advantage in your CV. Look at these examples:

Mary Jones trained as a massage therapist once her children started school. Her experience of dealing with fraught mothers and their offspring led her to take further training in baby massage. In addition to her practice, she now teaches massage at the XYZ Health Centre.

Paul Green was a violinist with a London orchestra. He became interested in complementary therapies when dealing with the aches and pains brought about by his professional life. This led him to train as a massage therapist and his former colleagues now benefit from his new skills.

Joanna Brown has just completed her full-time education and recently qualified as a beauty therapist. She has always taken pride in her own appearance and her interest in clothes and make-up led her to set up her own business. She is currently undertaking further training as a colour analyst.

Your CV should contain your:

- name
- address (as this is for other health professionals, not clients)
- phone number
- date of birth
- marital status
- details of training, including any work experience you may have had in that time
- work experience, with the most recent first

4

THE PROFESSIONAL PRACTITIONER

Working within a code of conduct

Your training school may well have given you a code of conduct, reflecting best working practice. If so, you will have an idea of what is expected of the professional therapist. Fundamentally, this should lead to the practitioner working for the highest good of the client. A good code will therefore include most or all of the following:

Towards clients:

- You should behave with integrity and professionalism.
- You should work for the highest good of those you treat.
- You must respect client confidentiality.
- You should not attempt to give treatment beyond your ability.
- You must not claim to cure medical conditions.
- You must refer clients to their doctors if you suspect serious ill health (and record that you have given this advice).
- You must not abuse their trust or cause them undue distress or embarrassment.
- You should show your clients the consideration that you yourself would expect to receive.
- You should provide a clean, hygienic environment for treatment.

Towards colleagues:

- You should behave with consideration, fairness, professionalism and integrity.
- You should not criticise them.
- You should not attempt to entice other people's clients to see you.

Towards the medical profession:

- Remember that the doctor remains responsible for the care of his/her patient.
- You must seek a doctor's consent if treating someone with a serious illness (and record that you have received it).
- If the doctor refuses consent you should not treat the patient.
- You should keep a doctor informed of the progress of the patient (in writing unless s/he specifies otherwise).
- You should try to foster good working relationships with doctors.

For your own protection:

- You must be adequately insured.
- You must keep comprehensive records on clients.
- You should maintain the highest possible standards of practice.
- You should keep up-to-date with advances in your therapy.
- You should not make exaggerated claims for your therapy either verbally, or in advertising or literature.
- If in doubt about treating anyone, you should seek appropriate advice.

Initial contact

The telephone is often your client's initial contact with you. Keep the following points in mind when dealing with client phone calls:

- By your telephone manner you will encourage or discourage potential clients.
- The initial call provides your main opportunity to decide if this caller is someone you wish to treat.
- You can learn a lot by the caller's manner towards you.
- You need to decide if it is appropriate for you to treat individual callers, or whether they should be referred elsewhere.
- By getting much of the case history over the phone, you may not need to spend so much time on it when the client comes to you.
- It is better to use the answering machine and return the call later than to undersell yourself when caught at an inconvenient time.

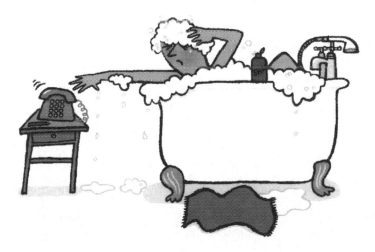

Your answering machine message should be businesslike, impersonal, but still welcoming. Do not give your name or any description of yourself (I answer the phone with my name, but I have a separate business line). Obtain as much information as possible from your client, including name, address and phone number. If you are uncertain that the caller is genuine, you could check further by calling them back to ask for further information for your records. Ask where the caller heard about you (this also helps you evaluate any advertising) and why he or she needs treatment.

If something about the caller rings your alarm bells, make an excuse not to treat the person however much you need the money.

If you make an appointment yet are still unhappy about someone coming to a clinic or to your home for the first time, either ensure that you are not alone with the client or ask a friend or colleague to phone you at a certain time while the client is there. Arrange a code to indicate to your friend whether or not you are safe. You can arrange the same if you are the one making the visit.

Creating the right impression

When working at home

Keep all doors shut except the one to your treatment room – no one will be impressed by the sight of your unmade bed! You may like to have some signs saying 'Private' or 'Toilet' on your doors. This gives the correct impression and minimises the opportunity for misunderstanding. You could leave a few children's toys around if you want to give the impression of having a family. Keep your personal appearance professional and businesslike.

The areas to which your clients have access need to be very clean and tidy (difficult for those of us with small children). Your treatment room and bathroom should be spotless.

Hygiene and appearance

On one course I attended, we were all told that, to avoid embarrassment, we would all be told the obvious about personal hygiene. I do the same here! No one receiving a treatment wants a lung-full of BO as you stretch across them! Daily washing and a change of underwear are essential for you. Nails should be kept clean and short. Your hair should be tidy and tied back if necessary. Jewellery is best kept to a minimum for those doing any kind of body work. Garlic, coffee breath, and cigarette smoke are completely antisocial, as is perfume!

Your appearance gives certain messages about you, so think carefully about what sort of image you intend to project. How formal or informal you look is up to you, but you need to look businesslike, clean and tidy. Remember that first impressions count for a lot.

Care of the client

You should have already learned the basic principles for the care of your client in the course of your training. However, it is such an important aspect that it is worth reminding ourselves of the following:

- Be welcoming and make your client feel at ease.
- Provide reassurance as to the nature of your treatment.
- Keep your clients covered to maintain their dignity as much as possible.
- Be sensitive to your clients' needs.
- Offer the use of a toilet.

In practice, care of your clients extends beyond the treatment room. They need your care as much before and after the treatment as during it. Your business is to make them feel valued.

Record keeping

Good record-keeping is essential for many reasons:

- Records provide the history of the client's medical condition.
- They remind us of the person's condition and what treatment we performed last time.
- They are a useful way of charting progress (people often forget the symptoms they came with, and our records help us to remind them once the symptoms have disappeared).
- We can record something we want to do or pick up on next session.
- They are useful for recording how often someone cancels or forgets appointments.
- They are useful to look back on in the event of a complaint.
- You won't remember everything about each client.

Records should contain at least the following:

- name, address and telephone number
- brief medical history
- any medication the client is taking
- the client's GP's name and address
- reason for treatment, such as relaxation/frozen shoulder/ depression
- symptoms at first consultation

Many people are poor historians. I ask all the pertinent questions. 'No,' the client replies, 'I've had no recent surgery.' I then find a large, livid scar, and when questioned the client says, 'Oh, that was my coronary artery bypass graft. I had it two months ago.' Or having told me that they have no musculo-skeletal problems, clients will get off the couch asking, 'Do you think this will help my bad back?'!!

I have been asked a couple of times by solicitors to write letters for patients claiming damages after a road traffic accident. I would not have been able to remember the details of dates, the number of treatments, or the progress of treatment, had I not kept detailed records of clients' visits.

Records should be kept in a safe place, preferably in a filing cabinet where they cannot be read by a casual observer.

The Data Protection Act 1998   If you keep any information on your clients' condition, diagnosis and details of treatment on computer, you will need to notify the Information Commissioner for the Data Protection Act.

However, if you keep all your records in a manual filing system, or the data kept on computer is restricted to name, address and payment details, then you are likely to be exempt. As legislation changes from time to time, it would be worth checking whether or not you need to register. There is a *Self Assessment Guide* on the Data Protection website, www.dpr.gov.uk. Further details are given in the address section of this book.

If the client is in ill health

If clients phone because they are ill and don't know whether to fulfil an appointment or not, what do you advise them? All the usual contra-indications apply, but the following questions can help too:

- Do they have a fever? (If so, tell them to stay at home.)
- Are they infectious? (If they are, you don't want their germs.)
- Is there any possibility that a treatment could exacerbate their condition? (If so, give the appointment a miss.)
- Do they actually want to be touched?
- Are you prepared to risk contracting their bug?

Reactions to treatment

The greatest darkness may well be unsupportable light.

Unknown

Those people used to allopathic medicine may be uncomfortable with the idea that it is possible to feel worse before feeling better. As we never know how someone will respond to treatment, it is worth mentioning that some form of reaction is perfectly normal. It is possible to do this without alarming your clients!

Some useful remedies for dealing with reactions to treatment:

- Arnica tablets for stiffness
- drinking lots of water to help excrete by-products of metabolism
- Rescue Remedy or Five Flower Essence if the client is feeling shaky
- reassurance
- a warm bath and a good night's sleep

If you have to cancel

Only the mediocre are always at their best.

Jean Giraudoux

For some unknown reason, many clients expect their therapists to be available, enthusiastic and healthy 24 hours a day, 365 days a year. Unfortunately, we cannot get away from the fact that sometimes we have to let clients down. If we cancel because we're ill, we let them down, but we let them down in an even worse way if we risk passing our germs on to them.

If you are unable to work for any reason, be it holiday or illness, it is responsible and professional to suggest a colleague who can cover for you. If your clients prefer to wait for you, that is fine, but at least you have given them the choice. I hear therapists voice concerns that their clients will desert them for whoever is covering. I can only say that I personally have never experienced a client doing this. I have passed my clients to colleagues during times of illness, holiday and maternity leave. My clients have been grateful for the chance to continue having massage while I was unavailable. It would seem that those who did *not* have treatment while their regular therapist was unavailable would be the ones to get out of the habit entirely, and never return for treatment.

If you do need to cancel appointments, be meticulous in ensuring that you contact those clients again afterwards. It can feel rather rejecting to have therapists promise to contact you when they're well again, only to never hear from them. It is also poor business management to lose clients because you are disorganised!

Dealing with other professionals

Your main contact with doctors and other health professionals is likely to be mostly by letter. Letters to all health professionals should be on headed notepaper. Write the letter in such a way that the other professional is likely to read it. I suggest you avoid using terms such as chakras, auras, energy blocks and the like, keeping your terminology as down-to-earth as possible. You are less likely to be dismissed as a New Age weirdo and have a better chance of the recipient taking notice!

If your letter relates to a particular patient, that person's name, address, and date of birth should be in bold after 'Dear Dr ——:'. You might like to remind the person you are writing to about the patient. Following are some sample letters:

Dear Dr Smith:

Penny White, 12 Green Street, Halifax.
DOB 4/11/50

I have now given several weekly treatments to this 48-year-old lady with rheumatoid arthritis. I have worked particularly on her painful feet, and the two swollen fingers on her left hand. I have carried out gentle passive joint movements to all her affected joints with the aim of improving her mobility.

She reports that she has less pain and is taking fewer analgesics. She is also able to take her dog for longer walks than previously. We are both pleased with her progress and I shall continue to treat her monthly from now on.

If you feel this is insufficient or would like further information, please do not hesitate to contact me.

Yours sincerely

As your business increases you may like to write as a

matter of course to your client's GP, if the client is willing to allow you. A standard letter to doctors could be something like this:

Dear Dr Bloggs:

Fred Smith, 12 The Green, Bloxwich.
DOB 8/6/60

I write as a matter of professional courtesy to inform you that your above-named patient has come to me for a course of massage treatment.

Massage can be beneficial in a number of complaints, particularly those which are stress-related. However, if you feel that massage is contra-indicated for this person, or you would like further information, please do not hesitate to contact me.

Yours sincerely

You should always seek a GP or hospital consultant's permission if your client is suffering from a serious medical condition, or has had recent surgery. If in doubt, you could arrange the client's appointment far enough ahead for you to do this. You may be asked to provide a CV or some information to show that you are competent. A doctor may also like to know that you are insured.

I have treated patients with active cancer, after recent open-heart surgery, after recent fractures, with severe neurological disease, even with a steel 'halo' following a neck fracture. In each case I have (usually) obtained written consent or (occasionally) verbal consent and I record this in the patient's notes. You should also notify the doctor of your client's progress. This is courteous to the doctor, and gives him or her some idea of the efficacy of your therapy.

Confidentiality

What does the issue of confidentiality actually mean to us as therapists? There are two important points to consider. One is that certain personal details pertaining to clients should never be revealed to anyone. For example, I do not write down information on such things as sexual abuse, violent relationships or rape. I write something which will remind me, but nothing which could be understood by anyone else.

The second point relates to the client's medical condition. It is sometimes helpful to discuss case histories with colleagues or other health professionals for the greater good of the patient. But the client should never be named in these discussions. If, however, you need to identify the client (for example, if you need to discuss treatment with the person's GP or other therapist) you must first ask for the client's permission. Even then, you might expect to discuss Miss Smith's bad back, but not the fact that she is currently in a violent relationship, even if you think this is relevant.

Handling difficult situations

Obscene phone calls

When ideas fail, words come in handy.

Goethe

The most obvious thing to say about obscene phone calls is that you do not have to listen to them! Most of us forget this when we pick up the phone and find ourselves with an obscene caller on the other end. If you do speak to the caller, make it plain exactly what you are offering, even saying that you do not offer any sexual services.

Aim to have separate business and private lines or a mobile phone as soon as you are able. You may find it useful to have a phone which displays the caller's number.

If nuisance calls become frequent, when you answer the phone, pause before you speak, then just say 'hello'. Do not argue, get angry or emotional. Rest the phone off the hook and go away, leaving the person talking. After a while, put the phone back on the hook *without* listening to hear if the caller is still there.

You can obtain information from British Telecom on dealing with malicious calls by dialling 150. If you are really worried, you can contact the BT recorded Advice Line on 0800 666700 or the BT Specialist Bureau on 0800 661441. You could also contact your local police community safety department. It is a criminal offence to make malicious calls and callers are liable to be prosecuted.

Erections during treatment

Remember that an erection is a perfectly normal physiological response. There is no need to overreact. Defuse the situation with a one-liner – sympathetic or not as appropriate. A full bladder can cause what looks like an erection, so before you make a withering comment, remember that the poor man may just be bursting for a wee!

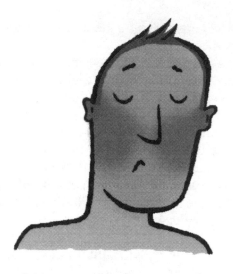

Sexual advances

If, during a treatment, a client makes sexual advances to you, end the session and make it clear that you are not interested. Ask the client to leave, without charging a fee. Have a ready-made excuse, for example, that your husband/wife is due home (even if you are unattached!). Do not compromise your professional integrity, however much you need the money. Provide yourself with a personal alarm or a panic button if you wish.

Weirdos

> **Good advice is a doubtful remedy, but generally not dangerous since it has so little effect.**
>
> Jung

It is natural for therapists to be concerned about possible encounters with violent or threatening people. Fortunately, this kind of problem is extremely rare. Many of

40

my colleagues have never felt unsafe or frightened. In my many years of practice I have had only one unpleasant experience. Although I was uneasy from the time of the initial phone call, I was foolish enough not to listen to the alarm bells ringing in my head! One thing is worth repeating – **If ever you are unhappy about treating someone, make an excuse and do not see the person.**

A group of therapists near me met with the police to discuss issues of personal safety. **Our conclusion was that the risk of violent confrontation is extremely rare.** If you think you will worry about this aspect of life as a therapist, however, consider taking lessons in self-defence or martial arts.

In the unlikely event that you find yourself in a difficult situation, remember the following:

- If possible, arrange beforehand for someone to phone or call at a pre-arranged time.
- Stay calm and defuse the situation rather than get angry.
- Do not compromise your professional integrity.
- Talk the experience through with a colleague afterwards.
- Learn from the experience and evaluate your handling of it.

Some therapists avoid this issue by treating persons of their own sex only. I personally feel that it is a pity to reject those seeking genuine treatment because of some vague potential risk. Sometimes a man's wife or secretary will phone to discuss an appointment. I like this, as I can also reassure myself about the client's intentions! If a man gives his name and phone number, in my experience he is genuine. Those seeking sexual services do not give their names, but enquire about the 'massage service'. You will soon learn to distinguish between the two kinds of callers, although you may still make mistakes. Occasionally I have stressed the fact that I do not provide sexual services, only to have some poor chap say, 'I'm gay', or 'But I've only got a bad shoulder!' However, it is better to risk offending a potential client than to end up in an unpleasant situation you could have avoided. Genuine enquirers will understand your position.

Smelly clients!

Occasionally you will encounter a client who has a real problem with personal hygiene. Dirty feet can be wiped with a baby wipe. Anyone can be a bit sticky on a hot day, but it is a brave therapist who cleans a client's underarms! You could suggest that less than fresh clients take a shower before you treat them, particularly if they wish to see you again!

Turning away a client

Love your neighbour but do not take down the fence.

Chinese proverb

What do you do if you form a violent aversion to someone who comes to you for treatment?

The answer depends on whether or not you can put your feelings on one side and give the client a good treatment while retaining your integrity and sanity. I don't believe it is necessary for me to like all those whom I treat, but it is vital to respect and tolerate them. I have one or two who have the effect of making my heart sink when I see their names in the diary. However, they must

42

feel they get a reasonable treatment or they would not come back for more!

It is very empowering to turn someone away occasionally. I once treated a lady with Multiple Sclerosis. She parked her car inconveniently for my neighbours (couldn't park well because of the MS). Then she demanded a drastically reduced fee (had no money because of the MS) and wanted an extra long treatment (because of the MS). Her appointment had to be at the same time each week (you'll have guessed why). She made offensive personal comments about my house (uninhibited because of MS). I finally ushered her out after two hours while she complained that I hadn't shown her any photos of my children. After she had gone I felt as if I had to brush bits of her off me! (More on dealing with other peoples' crud elsewhere.)

I dreaded her return, and eventually wrote to her saying that I felt I wasn't the right therapist for her and suggesting she find someone else.

If you do turn clients away, try to do it as gently as possible, but not so gently that they don't get the message!

First aid

There is nothing more frightening than a person collapsing in front of you, especially if you don't know what to do! The collapse may have nothing to do with the treatment you are offering, and to put the subject in context, I will say that I have witnessed more people collapsing in the supermarket than I have in my treatment room! However, it is sensible to have some knowledge of first aid. You could attend one of the courses run by either the British Red Cross Society or the St John's Ambulance Brigade. At least you should know how to deal with fainting, chest pain, asthma, cardiac arrest and cardio-pulmonary resuscitation.

Latecomers

It is also worth deciding what you will do about late-comers. My feeling is that your other clients who are on time should not be put out by those who are less punctual. Again, you should try to be flexible. If you have time to accommodate those who are late through no fault of their own, you should. But don't put your whole day out because of someone who is habitually late.

5

THE HUMAN TOUCH

Looking after yourself

Being is born of not being.
Lao Tsu, *The Tao Te Ching*

It is essential when looking after others that you also look after yourself. It goes without saying that if you advocate your therapy for others, you should practise what you preach and receive it yourself. Treating people can be very draining and you will need to recharge your batteries regularly. You also need to put your money where your mouth is when it comes to diet and exercise!

Availability

I cannot prevent the birds from flying overhead, but I can stop them nesting in my hair.
Chinese proverb

It is nine o'clock on Friday evening and you are pleasantly relaxed after a couple of glasses of wine. The phone rings – a potential new client is enquiring about an appointment. Do you answer the phone? Is your speech slurred? Do you sound coherent and can you sell yourself well? Will the client be put off by the fact that you have been drinking (conveniently forgetting that he or she rang at an intrusive time)?

It may be an automatic reaction to answer the phone, but your answering machine is your best ally on these occasions. I have had whole weeks when I would not have had an uninterrupted meal without the answering machine. I have also been phoned at 6 a.m. (by a farmer), at 11.30 p.m. (by a client who forgot to come that evening), in the middle of a dinner party (to change an appointment the following week), at 8.30 a.m. on New Year's Day, and on many other bank holidays.

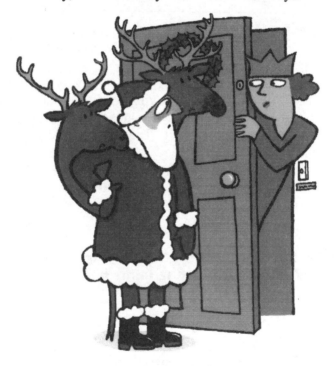

If you wish to reduce this kind of intrusion, it is worth telling your clients a good time to get hold of you. I deliberately do not return calls which I consider intrusive until the next day. You might like to leave a message on your answering machine as to when you can be contacted.

One of the disadvantages of working at home is that it is difficult to get away from your work. Make sure that you take regular holidays or short breaks. It is tempting to be too available when you first start out. You will become tired and stale if you don't ensure that you recharge your batteries regularly. (One of my rules is not to read professional papers or journals in the evening so that I avoid living and breathing massage.)

Equipment

I regard good equipment as part of looking after oneself. Ensure that your portable couch is easy to carry if you intend to do a lot of home visits. It is sensible to buy the best quality equipment that you can afford. It should then last you for years. Check that your car seats are comfortable if you will spend a lot of time travelling. Give some thought as to how you can best arrange your life so that, professionally, things go as smoothly as possible.

Crud (!)

Things fall apart, the centre cannot hold. Mere anarchy is loosed upon the world.
W.B. Yeats, *The Second Coming*

Most of us have experienced occasions when friends come round for a good moan. They feel marvellous afterwards, but we are left with the crud they have dumped on us! This situation is magnified when we treat clients, particularly in massage, where we have skin-to-skin contact.

It is generally accepted that we hold anger, distress and other emotions in our muscles. We are therefore highly likely to release these feelings during treatment. What do we do if we feel we are left with unpleasant emotions, or something triggers our own emotional excess baggage? I once heard a doctor describe this situation as 'emotional cross-infection'. Do we also risk cross-infecting our other clients emotionally if we do not take steps to avoid it?

Golden rules for avoiding others' crud:

- Protect yourself before touching anybody.
- Wear designated clothes for work and change when you have finished.
- Use clean towels and paper couch roll for each person.
- Open the window for fresh air between clients.
- Wash your hands in cold water between clients.
- Cleanse the room with incense/candles/crystals/flower essence.
- Take Rescue Remedy if needed.
- Always shower after you have finished (or visualise it if the real thing is impossible).
- If you suspect a client will upset you, take a few drops of Bach Flower Rescue Remedy, or Walnut Remedy if you need psychic protection.

Psychic protection

The best lack all conviction, while the worst are full of passionate intensity.
W.B. Yeats, *The Second Coming*

It is difficult to talk about psychic protection without sounding mysterious or airy-fairy. However, it is such an important aspect of therapeutic work that I mention it and leave you to formulate your own personal protection. Most of the successful therapists I know seem to have some form of protection ritual, and something to cleanse themselves afterwards.

Much depends on your beliefs and sensitivities. The

48

simplest protection is to imagine yourself enveloped in a huge ball of white light through which nothing negative can penetrate. Judy Hall in her book *The Art of Psychic Protection* suggests stepping into a hoop of light which you can pull up around you. She also has some wonderful images of psychic laser guns and vacuum cleaners to remove any lingering nasties.

I had one client, later diagnosed as schizophrenic, who was very difficult and disturbed. I used to visualise myself in a diving bell so that I could treat him without problems. I also visualise the spider plant in my treatment room soaking up any negativity.

If I feel that my treatment room is harbouring anything negative, I mentally sweep the room, open the window wide and allow the crud to fall into a large psychic

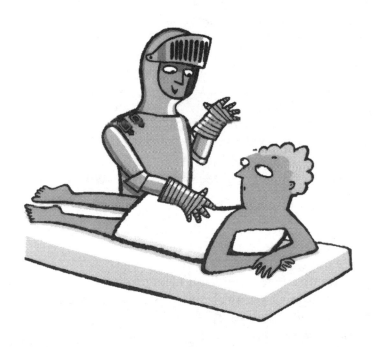

'sludge gulper' lorry which sits outside my house while I work. The lorry leaves after I have finished and returns the next time I need it. You can also 'smudge' a room with American Indian Smudge sticks.

Your own stuff

I would know my shadow and my light, so shall I at last be whole.
                    Sir Michael Tippett, *A Child of our Time*

Occasionally when someone confides in me, I am left feeling distressed by their revelations. Showering and changing my clothes is a useful ritual for shedding the day's distress. If that fails, I take Rescue Remedy or Star of Bethlehem. I always burn a joss stick at the end of every day as part of my ritual. (It is good for getting rid of cooking smells too.) Remember that colleagues can be supportive when you need them. Sometimes all you need is a massage yourself or a friendly ear.

Give yourself a time limit for dealing with distress. If you are no better by your self-imposed deadline, seek professional help. If you have done a good job of making contacts, you will know a psychotherapist or counsellor who will be able to help. If you think I am exaggerating the need for psychic protection and dealing with crud, here is a list of some of the things I have had divulged to me:

- rape (at least two, including that of a 9-year-old)
- sexual abuse (four or five cases)
- violent relationship (several)
- death of client's child/ren (several)
- client sent to prison (he claims to be innocent)
- suicide of client's son
- messy divorce

50

- severe psychiatric illness and/or depression
- post-traumatic stress disorder

If several of these crop up in a short space of time, you can feel pretty chewed up. In order to remain effective as a therapist and human being, you need to find ways of coping with and processing your distress. Counsellors are obliged to have regular supervision in order to work well. As there is no obligation upon complementary therapists to do that, I suggest you find your own appropriate form of support and care, preferably *before* you need it.

This helps *you* to cope, but what about the poor client? Most of us are not trained counsellors and do not have the necessary skills to deal with such traumas. It is important that we acknowledge the client's distress while making it clear that we cannot help. I say something like 'I can see this is very distressing for you. Have you thought of whom you might go to to talk about it?' I then suggest a referral to a colleague who has the skills to help.

I leave this subject with a quote.

> Caring persons must be prepared to suffer within the suffering of others. We shall only be able to do this when we have enough health within ourselves to be able to continually expose ourselves to the person in need of care. As we search for a deeper and greater awareness of our own emotional and spiritual needs, I would suggest that only in our growing awareness of these needs, dare we enter into the sufferings of others. Dare we ask the other person the real reason for his suffering? Dare we ask what this suffering is doing and/or means? Dare we communicate in such a manner as to enable him and ourselves to grow through his suffering, our mutual

51

suffering? Caring persons are not healers, at best they are *enablers of healing*.' [my italics]

From an article in *Nursing Times*, 1980

Client needs

Men are cruel but man is kind.

Rabindranath Tagore

In view of the above, I would suggest that our clients' greatest need is for us to be gentle with them. We often don't know what has happened to people, and they often do not reveal their distress immediately. Only once has someone walked into my treatment room and said, 'Hello, I'm Jenny and I've been sexually abused.' It is more usual for them to come for treatment for a long time (years rather than months) before saying anything. The same goes for those whose children have died, those who have been raped or are in violent relationships. Some people are very conscious of being overweight. ('I'll just lose another stone before I come to you.') Others have had other kinds of traumatic experiences which require gentle handling.

We need to be aware of our potential to hurt our clients unintentionally. If you insist that someone removes her underwear for a treatment and she has had a sexual trauma in the past, aren't *you* being abusive? I think it is better to give a less thorough treatment than to cause a client distress.

Remember too, that a client may have suffered at the hands of another therapist. After I had given evidence in a court case against a colleague (who was convicted of sexual assault), some of his victims said that they missed having massage, but felt too vulnerable to try again.

I once went to a colleague for a massage. I made it clear that I was tired and wanted to drift off during the treatment. I also said I was very upset, having just heard that a friend had been diagnosed with cancer. When I said he only had 15 years maximum to live, her response was 'That's good. Most people die of cancer much quicker than that.' She then spent the massage chatting, asking me about my husband's job, and telling me how sensitive she is!

Apart from gentleness and acceptance, what else do our clients need? I believe those needs vary from treatment to treatment. Sometimes clients need silence, sometimes to talk, sometimes a gentle rub, sometimes a vigorous workout. You should develop sensitivity to your client's needs over time. You can always reflect back your own perceptions: 'I sense you need a gentle massage today, is that right?' Ask open questions such as 'How are you feeling ?' or 'Is this what you want today?'

If you chat too much during the massage, you are taking your client's time rather than him or her taking yours. A certain amount of chat is fine, as your clients may want to get to know you. Just be aware that too much can become unhealthy.

I remember having Alexander Technique lessons with a woman who (ab)used her clients. It was impossible to concentrate while she related the gruesome details of her abortion/divorce/violent relationship. Several of my friends had lessons from her too, and we all had the same experience and the same tale of woe. She had no idea of what she was doing to her clients, even telling us off if we didn't get something right! (I should say that I have since had Alexander Technique lessons with really professional, caring people.)

Sometimes outside influences prevent us from doing our best. One day I was treating a lady I'd been seeing for a couple of years. She was just confiding that she had been sexually abused by a relative when my new washing machine arrived unexpectedly! Fortunately, I was able to give her more time after the washing machine had been installed.

On another occasion I treated someone when I was completely exhausted. The tears were pouring down my face by the end of the session. I was just about to say that I thought my client should not pay me for such a poor treatment when she said, 'That was one of the best massages you've ever given me. It was really grounded and calm.' It would seem that even when we are feeling less than our best, we can help others. I have talked to colleagues about this, and many have felt on occasion that a treatment they gave was no good. The client has then declared it to be excellent! I believe that this may happen because of our intention for our clients (see later).

I need you NOW

The main thing in life is not to be afraid to be human.

Pablo Casals

It is difficult when someone rings wanting treatment NOW. You will have to judge each situation on its merits and decide whether or not you are being taken for granted. Remember that inflammation and some acute conditions are contra-indications for massage. It may be preferable for the person to use an ice pack, and to take pain relief until the acute condition subsides. The client should also consult a doctor or osteopath as appropriate.

Late one Christmas Eve, I was phoned by a man I'd never met who wanted a treatment NOW. He had ignored his condition which had been getting worse for months, finally catching up with him at Christmas. As it happened I was waiting for a doctor to visit my child who was ill, so it was easy to say no. The man tried a few other numbers I gave him (without success) and came to me afterwards at a more convenient time.

Of course there will be occasions when you will be happy to put yourself out for your clients, but do think carefully about it first. You may have ambitions to heal the sick and change the world, but you cannot be effective 24 hours a day, 365 days a year. It is important to take regular holidays and to have enough rest yourself. After all, this is what you would probably advise your clients to do!

To refuse clients at inconvenient times, I usually say that massage is a strenuous job and they would not receive a good treatment from me at 11 p.m. or whatever they have asked for. Or that if they had phoned at 2 p.m. instead of 6 p.m., I could have seen them that day.

This is where you can cooperate with other therapists. Find out when your colleagues are working, and let them know your hours. You can then help by giving each other's phone numbers if you are unable to treat someone.

6

SUPPORT GROUPS AND CONTINUOUS TRAINING

Imagine yourself alone in the midst of nothingness and then try to tell me how large you are.
Eddington

Complementary therapy support groups have a number of things to offer the newly qualified therapist:

- They help you to meet other therapists.
- Other therapists get to know you.
- They provide stimulation of new ideas and professional development.
- They offer support that helps reduce isolation.
- They sometimes print lists of therapists, helping to generate work.
- They give you a chance to make friends/swap treatments.
- They help keep you up-to-date with developments in your therapy.

What do you do if there is no support group in your area? Start one! If you don't feel up to organising a big group, you could get together with a few therapists. If your home is not suitable, you could meet at a pub or village hall. When I first embarked on setting up a support group, I was surprised and delighted by the friendly, positive response I received from other therapists.

The group I started grew to about 30 therapists who met four times a year. Some of the group have become really close friends and I value them greatly. We had a mixture of meetings with speakers, and social occasions. Therapists also swap skills. For example, one person with computer skills does a job in exchange for another therapist's essential oils. Therapists new to the area could find out about work possibilities and feel less isolated. We produced a list of therapists which we distributed to health food shops, leisure centres, dentists, libraries and anywhere else we could. The initial work of setting up our group was well worth the effort.

Further training and updating skills

We shall either find what we are seeking, or free ourselves from the persuasion that we know what we do not know.

Socrates

You may feel that the last thing you want to consider now is further training. But it is essential that you keep up-to-date in your therapy and gain stimulation from new ideas. Further training need not mean lengthy, expensive courses. It is possible to find one-day workshops or evening lectures to interest you. Some support groups put on excellent talks by knowledgeable speakers. While you are less busy, use your time to read about your subject and consolidate your knowledge. (Once you become busy, there may not be enough time for this.) You should also consider subscribing to a relevant journal. Occasional visits to health exhibitions can be useful. Your training school may be glad of your help if it is taking part. It may also give study days, conferences and workshops.

As regulation of complementary therapies becomes a stronger possibility, your training school or umbrella organisation may require you to complete a statutory amount of study each year.

7

MONEY

Abundance and attitudes to money

> On your quest for abundance think of the symbology of the woodpecker. Each peck does not amount to much but eventually the whole bloody tree comes down.
>
> Stuart Wilde, *The Trick to Money is Having Some*

There are plenty of books available on the subject of abundance which can help you explore your attitude to money. It is worth doing so; it is easy to believe that we are free from prejudice and fixed ideas until we look closely!

I emphasise again that if you are offering something of value, you deserve to be paid accordingly. Even healers need to eat and pay the rent or mortgage. Some therapists like to have another part-time job. This helps relieve anxiety about any lack of clients in quiet times, while paying some bills.

Setting fees

> Learning to charge properly is a vital key to abundance. Affirm that you will never devalue yourself by charging less than what you feel you are worth.
>
> Stuart Wilde, *The Trick to Money is Having Some*

I receive more requests for advice on this than anything else, so it obviously causes a few headaches. If you pitch your fees very low, you are undervaluing your therapy and yourself. You will upset your colleagues who charge a more realistic rate, and potential clients may be suspicious of someone so cheap. Be clear that you are offering something of value for which you deserve to be paid an appropriate fee. One client thought my fees were high, as she could have massage elsewhere much more cheaply. She phoned me some weeks later to say that the cheaper massage was nowhere near as good as mine, so she would prefer to come to me in the future.

You should review your fees annually. You may not wish to increase them each year, but you should make a conscious decision about it.

Points to consider:

- What is the going rate locally? (Ring round to find out.)
- Will you offer a reduced rate when you first start?
- If so, for how long before raising your fees?
- How many free treatments are you prepared to give?
- What do you consider to be your value (in terms of what you offer in a treatment)?
- What outgoings will you have to cover?
- Will you charge extra for home visits?
- What sort of attitude do you have to money?

Free treatments

You pay me for my time. The healing comes free.
Matthew Manning, healer

When starting out, it is good to be prepared to give some free treatments. However, you should think about how many, and for how long you will do this. People often do not appreciate what they get for nothing, and sometimes a token payment is more appropriate. When I began, I gave someone a lot of free treatments. She would always say, 'What a shame you can't have massage as often as me.' I would feel really resentful because if she had paid me, I could have had!

When I first started working as a therapist, I gave a free treatment to someone who then recommended me to a friend of hers. The friend passed my phone number to a lot of people and my business grew substantially as a result. It was really worth my while to give that free treatment. The important thing is that both you and the client are happy with the arrangement and that you do not feel taken for granted.

Some choices are to:

- Give the first treatment free, then charge your normal fee for further treatments.
- Give some free treatments as appropriate, but review the situation after you have given a few.
- Offer, for example, 12 treatments for the price of 10 (paid in advance).
- Barter   the client performs a service for you in return for treatment (though your accountant will not like it).

Reducing Fees

Misfortune is an occasion to show character.
                                                    Seneca

You will undoubtedly be asked from time to time to reduce your fees for someone. The important issue here, as with free treatments, is that you are comfortable with the arrangement and do not feel taken for granted. It is perfectly acceptable to say no! After all, you need to pay your bills just like everyone else, and you deserve to be paid for what you do.

I went to massage a man in his own home. Once I gained admission at the electronic gates, a servant took my couch upstairs, past the enormous swimming pool, into the gymnasium. I was amazed when the client asked me to reduce my fees, but he accepted with good grace when I refused. I suspect that this was some sort of ritual which he felt obliged to go through. (I later learned that he owned a chain of extremely smart hotels in central London.) In another case, a therapist friend of mine reduced her fees after hearing a client's sob story. One day she happened to drive past the client's house. When she saw the expensive cars, the stable block and swimming pool, resentment set in!

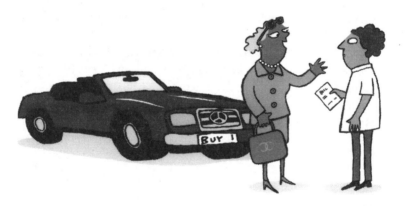

You will have to judge each case on its individual merits, but do beware of taking on other peoples' poverty. I have been given some amazing reasons for why I should accept reduced fees, including clients going on safari, going on holiday, going to the theatre, buying a new car, having three horses to feed, and paying for a child to attend a private school.

Whether or not you reduce fees depends on how much you want to see a particular client. You may decide to reduce fees for no one; if clients can't pay for your services, they need not come. But if you do decide to reduce fees, you have several options:

- Reduce for a short time agreed upon by both you and the client.
- Reduce for a client who introduces another client.
- Offer a 'standby' rate for a short notice appointment.
- Reduce long-term treatment fees by a small amount.

Cancellations

Unless you are to suffer a great deal of inconvenience, it is essential to have a policy on cancellations. I experienced a lot of short notice cancellations until I told all my clients that I reserved the right to charge for them. You will soon get to know who is taking you for granted, and you are likely to feel resentful towards them unless you take action! In practice, however, you will probably need to be flexible. If someone has crashed a car on the way to you, or a relative has died suddenly, you may be prepared to waive the cancellation fee. But if clients just forget, you may want to charge them. Clients will sometimes offer to pay anyway, as they then no longer feel under an obligation to you.

Some therapists charge a half fee for cancellations with less than 48 hours' notice and a full fee for 24 hours' notice. It may be worth printing something in your brochure about your policy. Remember, it is much easier to waive a cancellation fee than to ask for one from a client who doesn't expect it.

Reluctant payers

If people value what you do for them, they will pay you, as they will want to see you again. However, occasionally it is necessary to chase a client for payment. It is useful to have a computer for typing and keeping a record of your bills. In over 10 years of practice I have never had a bounced cheque, and very rarely had to write off payment. I have written off a few cancellations, but this is more commonly an area of negotiation between the therapist and client. It is easier to take payment at the end of the consultation than to send out a bill. If a potentially awkward situation develops, address it quickly before it gets out of hand.

8

ACCOUNTS AND TAXATION

It is better to light one small candle than to rail against the dark.

Gandhi

Type of business

When you start out in business as a complementary therapist you may be:

- an employee (for example working for someone else at a health farm)
- in partnership (working together with a colleague)
- self-employed (you work for yourself, either from home or at a health clinic)

Employees will work a set number of hours in a room provided by their employer; they will be provided with the equipment they need for their job, and receive a regular income including holiday and possibly sickness pay. Theirs is the most straightforward situation. Their income is assured for as long as they remain employed. They do not need to keep business accounts and their employer should deduct income tax and National Insurance from their weekly or monthly income. If they have no other sources of income, they will not even have to complete a tax return (unless asked to do so by the Inland Revenue)!

A few therapists may start their practice in partnership with a friend or colleague. Others may also join the partnership once their practices have started. Legal advice should be sought before the partnership begins in order to establish the basis on which the partners will act. It follows that it is vital to choose the right partner from the outset. The partnership will be required to keep detailed accounts, with all partners reporting their share of the profits on their tax return.

Many complementary therapists work on a self-employed basis where they are in business on their own account. These individuals are ultimately responsible for how the business is run and are in control of what they do, and when, how and where they provide treatment. Their income may fluctuate but they will receive all the benefits from the growth of their business over time. Self-employed people will have to keep detailed accounts of their income, expenditure and assets, and must complete a tax return each year.

Keeping accounts

Whether you are self-employed or in partnership, you must keep detailed accounts and supporting records. It is well worth speaking to an accountant at an early stage of setting up in business, as it is much harder to put the records together once you have been working for a while. The key documents which you should keep are:

- a ledger to record all business income and business expenditure
- receipts for any business expenditure incurred
- a copy of any invoices issued
- bank statements

- cheque book stubs
- appointments diary

You should keep these records for at least six years after the end of the tax year.

A ledger is 'accountant speak' for a book in which you write all the receipts on the left-hand side and all the expenses on the right. For each item of income, identify the client who paid you and the date. For each item of expenditure, record to whom it was paid and what it was for, so that you can show that it was a business expense. If you like using computers, there are many software packages that will help you do the job. However, you will still need to find some time each week, if not each day, to keep your accounts up-to-date.

The kind of things you should be able to claim as business expenses are:

- stationery, business cards, brochures, postage
- books and subscriptions to professional journals
- insurance costs
- special clothing
- further training and associated costs such as travel, parking, some meals
- secretarial assistance
- advertising
- bank charges associated with a business loan
- any equipment such as couch covers, towels, oils
- computer costs if used exclusively for work

If you are working from home you may also be able to claim a proportion of:

- your household fuel bills for heat and light and laundry

- your telephone/mobile phone call costs, excluding the standing charge
- your car expenses if you use it for home visits

It is better to bank all money earned, cash as well as cheques, even if you then need to withdraw money as a separate transaction. Cash is otherwise untraceable. By paying it all in, you can correlate your income with your diary. Do not be tempted to 'lose' payments in cash. It is far better to be legal and above board in your financial affairs. Cash businesses are more prone to close scrutiny by the Inland Revenue!

Each year you will have to produce a summary of your income and expenditure in order to produce a record of your profit (or loss) for the year and the assets used in the business. Depending on your own skills and interest, you may wish to find an accountant who specialises in dealing with small businesses to help with this stage. Most charge by the hour (my accountant jokes that it's actually by the minute!), so you will reduce the cost if you have kept your own books on a regular basis and retained all the supporting documents listed above.

Income tax

Self-employed individuals and partners are required to complete a tax return for each year. For historic reasons, the tax year runs from 6 April to 5 April. Your accounts can, however, run to any date as long as it is consistent from one year to the next – say 31 December each year. Your income tax liability for the tax year 2002/2003, for example, will then be based on the profits earned by your business in the year ended 31 December 2002 – the accounts that end in the tax year.

If your gross income is less than £15,000, you need only submit a summary of your profits to the Inland Revenue. Where they are more than that, more detailed accounts are required. In either case, your tax liability will be based on your income earned, less expenses incurred for the accounts year. At this stage some expenditure will not be allowed as a deduction for tax purposes (for example, expenditure incurred entertaining professional contacts or suppliers over lunch). Also, if you spend money on something which will last a long time (over 2 years) such as a couch, other professional equipment or a computer, you may not get a deduction immediately. The tax system generally allows small businesses to claim a capital allowance equal to 40% of the cost in the first year and then 25% of the reduced balance each subsequent year. For example, if you spend £1000 on equipment, you can claim a deduction of £400 in the first year, £150 in the second year ((£1000–£400) x 25%), and so on. It can take about ten years to claim the full deduction of the original £1000. However, the Chancellor periodically introduces higher allowances on some types of equipment. It is worth checking each year whether you can claim any higher allowances.

You will be able to deduct your personal allowance from your profits each year. Amounts remaining will then be taxed at the rates set by the government. If you submit your tax return by 30 September each year, the Inland Revenue will calculate the amount of tax that you owe. Otherwise you will have to do it yourself and submit the return by 31 January. It is important that you submit your return no later than 31 January if you wish to avoid an automatic £100 penalty. Penalties increase for further delays and higher penalties are applied if returns are submitted late for three consecutive years.

Unlike the system for employees where tax is deducted

from their pay packet each week/month, the self-employed practitioner pays tax on 31 July and 31 January each year. Careful planning is required to make sure that you have the funds available as interest will be incurred on any tax which is paid late.

This is merely a summary of the main principles. You will almost certainly need advice in this area and should seek the assistance of your accountant.

National Insurance

Contact your local Benefits Agency when you start your business in order to organise your National Insurance contributions. This should be done within three months. If your income exceeds £4,025 (for 2002/2003) you are obliged to pay a class 2 stamp at a fixed rate per week of £2.00 (for 2002/2003). These can be paid by monthly Direct Debit. You will also have to pay a class 4 stamp equal to 7% of your income above £4,615 (for 2002/2003). This is paid with your income tax liability.

The payments entitle you to basic sickness pay, maternity pay, and your state pension. The state payments from these are not large, so you may well wish to insure yourself against the risks separately. (See chapter on insurance.)

Pension

If you wish to retire with a pension other than that offered by the state, you will need to put some money aside for the future. At present tax reliefs are available for contributions to pension funds. However, there are many ways of saving for the long term and also many providers in the market. You would therefore be well advised to discuss your options with an independent financial adviser before making any commitment.

9

INSURANCE

Although Insurance is something many people distrust or simply don't understand, it is vital when running a Practice to consider your package of protection and support against any possible financial vicissitudes in life. Insurance has offered valuable protection and support to many people for a very long period of time, and should be carefully considered, so that the same thoughtfulness and quality choices are made as in other areas of your practice. Although this chapter may be a useful guide, there is no substitute for a skilled advisor preferably specialising in Insurance for Health Professionals, who can customise your package to suit your individual circumstances

Insurance is not only for the protection of you, the practitioner, but also for your patients and the general public. Insurance is an essential factor in any business and is particularly relevant to practitioners in their contact with patients. Indeed, it is an integral aspect of professionalism and is particularly important in the current climate of greater recognition. More and more people are turning towards other approaches to health and healing, leading to greater exposure, and consequently a greater possibility of situations occurring or allegations of negligence against practitioners taking place.

With the advent of 'no win, no fee' solicitors, it easier than before to pursue a legal case. There are also disciplinary and complaint avenues for the public, which, since Statutory Regulation, is beginning to be used more and more.

Furthermore, there is the ongoing harmonisation in the practice of Natural Medicine within the Single European Market. The Government bodies want to see Complementary Medicine getting more professional and less fragmented, either through self-regulation or statutory regulation (such as osteopaths, chiropractors etc). There is a move towards greater quality control in areas of training standards, codes of conduct, ethics and insurances. In the past, insurance was seen as a necessary evil, or even not considered important at all, especially by a number of practitioners who relied on the fact that their type of therapy was safe or that they had never had a claim in their career, or simply because they did not philosophically believe in it! Clearly this degree of naivety is no longer tenable or acceptable to the wider Institutional world.

We will now explore some of the principal types of Insurance that are relevant to you in setting up your practice, and protecting it against unforeseen mishaps which may arise!

Working from Home? Household Insurance considerations

The standard householders policy will cover the building of your home or the contents for specific perils like fire, lightning, storm damage, overflowing of water, explosion, earthquake, aircraft, riot and civil commotion, malicious damage, theft and subsidence. Most policies offer an extension for accidental damage, to cover such things as staining, breaking, tearing, and scratching insured items. A word of warning for the practitioner; the

73

standard house policy is intended for a home which is occupied residentially. Many insurance policies will not provide cover where there is business use, especially not if members of the public are routinely coming in. Some insurers take the view that if the house is used for business purposes, the risk is changed and may well be increased. It is vital that insurers are advised of business use so that they cannot repudiate a claim because they were not informed.

It is very important that you advise your insurer and preferably obtain a satisfactory response in writing. There are now a number of policies which combine Home and Business covers, but check these out before buying. They can be a little inflexible and can be more expensive than a specialist Surgery policy plus ordinary Household Insurance combination.

Surgery/Practice Room Combined Packages

These policies cover the general contents of the practice for perils such as those for Household Insurance above for your furniture, equipment and stock. Typically, the first £50, £100 or even £250 may not be covered. This is known as the 'policy excess'. There may be expensive and delicate items of equipment in your clinic. These might be accidentally damaged, e.g. knocked over or broken. You need to ask your insurer for wider accidental damage cover if you possess any such equipment.

These policies also provide various other covers, such as Public Liability and Employers' Liability, detailed below.

This Insurance should also cover you for the loss of money in notes, coins and cheques on or off the premises for specific amounts. Loss of Profits or increased Cost of Working cover following property or contents damage, where the practice room is rendered unusable, and other optional covers, such as All Risks for items in transit, or temporarily removed can be covered.

Employer's Liability

If you employ other staff, it is a legal requirement that you effect employer's liability insurance. An employer's liability policy will meet the cost of any damages or other legal costs incurred where you, as the employer, have been held to be liable in some way.

Typically, an employee could claim that the premises were unsafe or injury had been caused by the equipment in the clinic. Your policy will only provide cover if you are legally liable but there will be a generous limit of indemnity of £10 million for any one incident. If a payment is made to an employee, the damages awarded will relate to the seriousness of the injury and financial loss of the employee. Most Surgery Packages include this, as mentioned above.

Public Liability

Public liability is simply an insurance to protect the practitioner against a claim from a member of the general public and such policies usually have a limit of £1 million for any one payment. It is also known colloquially as 'trip and slip' cover. If a patient were to trip over your carpet or fall down the stairs, he or she might be seriously injured. If a member of the public got hurt the practitioner could be sued for an allegation of negligence. A public liability policy enables the practitioner to sleep peacefully at night, knowing that he or she would be fully protected if such an unfortunate and unforeseen accident occurred. You have a responsibility to make sure that your premises are safe and any potentially hazardous items should not be left lying around. The same applies if you rent rooms at a Complementary Medicine Health Centre. Although the owner may say that they have Public Liability Cover, this will protect them if they are deemed legally liable, but not you. For example, you might be accused of damaging the room in some way, or your patient may be injured as a result of something you have done, so please don't rely on someone else's policy to protect you, as a number of practitioners sometimes do!

Public Liability with Treatment Risk Extension

In the early days of specialist natural medicine insurance, the majority of policies to protect practitioners from claims were somewhat restricted in scope. Of these the general public liability insurance with a treatment risk extension tagged on to it were the most commonly available. Additionally, some types of scheme may only cover one of a limited range of therapies. Practitioners who practise two or more therapies may find that they have to pay extra for the additional disciplines practised. Public liability with a treatment risk extension is often only valid either whilst the practitioner is treating, prescribing or advising a patient and normally covers the practitioner for incidents occurring in the year insured. A major disadvantage is that they cannot be upgraded in future years, to safeguard the practitioner for any (as yet) undiscovered claims, which may surface at a time when court awards are rising. These can sometimes leap up due to changes in case law, changes in interest rates for Settlement Damages Cash Awards that are invested plus the fact that inflation has gradually eroded the value of the indemnity limit (typically £500,000 or £1,000,000) which applied to the year when the treatment took place.

76

Professional indemnity

In this day and age, the treatment risk extension is simply not adequate. The general public are much more aware of their rights and will sue a practitioner if the treatment they have received has in any way caused them injury, pain or suffering, or if there is a pure financial loss, allegation of Breach of Confidentiality, etc. In an era of increasing competition amongst therapists, allegations of libel or slander may arise not only made by patients or clients, but also from other practitioners or teachers.

Under the Statute of Limitation, if someone wishes to sue you, they have to initiate proceedings within a 3-year period for injury claims after the date of discovery or 6 years for damage or financial loss claims. In the case of a minor, these limits apply after the age of majority (18).

Practitioners can now opt to cover their professional indemnity and malpractice insurance at a relatively inexpensive price. While covers used to be expensive, the growth of the natural medicine market has ensured a more competitive marketplace and specialist covers have been developed.

A professional indemnity insurance is practitioner based rather than therapy based. A good policy should insure the practitioner for full professional indemnity risks as well as public liability referred to above and product cover referred to later. The policy should cover more than one clinic where appropriate, and be flexible enough to include all of your therapies. The insurers normally require copies of certificates or qualifications and the premium will be based on classification of risk and the number of therapies. Premiums for therapies involving manipulation will be more expensive than for counselling.

Unlike most policies you may be familiar with, which provide cover for the damage at the time it occurs, professional indemnity policies provide cover at the time when a potential claim is reported to or discovered by the practitioner. Thus a current policy would provide cover in respect of treatment carried out some years previously but when the client has only now reported injury.

It is important when you effect a malpractice policy to agree with the insurers the number of years that you have been practising, for which they will now meet a claim. The technical term is 'the retroactive date'. When you terminate the policy you will need to arrange 'run-off' cover to ensure that your protection is ongoing, and can be revised from year to year, until you are clear of the statute of limitation period. Many of the best policies currently available automatically include these clauses.

You should also appreciate that liability and indemnity policies normally only cover civil liability or negligence. Allegations of Criminal Negligence or allegations of sexual impropriety for example, would not be covered unless you have a specialist Legal Cover for these types of situation.

What can I do to lessen the likelihood of a complaint or successful action against me for malpractice?

Here are some relevant points and a few basic precautions you can take to avoid situations occurring:

(a) Do not display your Insurance Certificate on the wall; for some people, it may be an open invitation to claim, and you could be prejudicing your Insurers.

(b) Policy conditions state you should make Patient Records and keep them for 7 years. We would suggest that you keep them longer than that, particularly in respect of child patients, where the Statute of Limitation states that a claim could be brought against you for injury cases up to 3 years after reaching the age of majority.

78

(c) Your patient notes are a main source of defence –
make sure that they are intelligible to others and
always keep them in a safe place, preferably locked.
Avoid assumptions or inferences and stick to observed
facts. Any alterations if in your own hand should be
crossed out and initialled/dated. Confidentiality and
Data Protection Issues should always be considered.

(d) You must notify your Brokers within 30 days of any
circumstance which may give rise to any claim.
Always declare previous incidents on any forms you
have to complete when starting or renewing cover,
even though you think the underwriter may already
know about them. Do not enter into dialogue or
correspondence about the complaint. Insurers may
decline a claim if you do not comply with policy
terms and conditions.

(e) Take care when advertising and in conversation, that
no claims for cure are made. Even anecdotal con-
versations about your previous successes may be
interpreted wrongly.

(f) A number of complaints seem to flow from misun-
derstandings or communications issues, and a failure
to establish a good quality therapeutic relationship.

(g) Refer when appropriate; particularly if a condition or
situation is beyond the scope of what you have been
trained to do, or where you may feel out of your depth.

(h) Extra care needs to be taken with child patients,
particularly where they may be experiencing headaches or high temperatures.

(i) If you are a multitherapist, and you decide to employ
a different therapy from the one that your patient
came for, involve the patient in that decision and
ensure that your patient is in agreement. Make sure
that the patient notes reflect this process and can be
followed.

(j) For techniques involving contact in erogenous zones, make sure that you have explained this and obtained patient's permission, preferably written, and/or offer a chaperone. Record this in the notes.

How do you recognise a Professional Indemnity or Medical Malpractice Claim?

Many situations can be regarded as potential claims, before they actually become formal claims made against you, either directly in writing, or via a solicitor. It is important that the warning signs are noticed, and acted upon as soon as possible to reduce the chances of a claim developing further, with the consequent stress and possible effect on your reputation. It is understood that you may not be negligent – the cover is there to help you clear your name if innocent, or deal with the expenses and costs if you are found negligent.

Danger signs include:

- Verbal complaint from a dissatisfied patient or client, with a threat of taking things further.
- Letter of complaint alleging dissatisfaction, neglect, error or omission.
- A patient not showing up for a subsequent treatment without explanation or further contact.
- A client or patient refusing to settle or delaying settlement of your account for an unreasonable period.
- A request for a refund of fees because the treatment has not worked or met with expectations, or is stated as having caused harm in some way

What should I do if a patient complains?

- Try not to panic or get defensive. Maintain goodwill.

Above all, *do not admit liability or indicate that you are insured. Your position will get weakened and it will make it more difficult for the insurers to successfully defend you.* Remember you must notify your insurers once you become aware of any situation, which may possibly result in a claim being made against you.

- If the incident involves any possible Criminal Proceedings you should phone your Legal Helpline, if your policy has one.
- Do not make any offers, but contact your intermediary (and the Helpline if appropriate).
- Do not try to defend yourself or get involved in correspondence or communications on your own account. Tactfully explain that you will reply when you have had time to consider the complaint further.
- Some surgeries have an in-house complaints procedure. This is a sign of good practice, but the procedure must be allowed to go hand in hand with your insurers' agreement at every stage.
- Pass on any correspondence received unanswered. Send in your patient notes and your response to the allegations.
- Try not to make any judgements as to whether the circumstances are valid or not, leave that to the Insurers or their representatives.
- If in doubt – notify!

Product Liability Insurance

If you make up or simply supply any of your own or other people's products or remedies (such as ointments, creams, aromatherapy or herbal prescriptions), you should ensure your policy provides product liability cover. This covers any legal liability following injury caused to anyone *as a result of a defect* in the product or remedy. Any incorrect advice causing injury or damage emerging from the advice is covered under the Malpractice or Treatment Risk Policy. Under the EC directive, you are held liable even if you innocently supplied the defective product. Some policies only cover you whilst supplying your own patients. If you retail these goods to people who are not your patients, you may need to arrange a separate policy.

10

PERSONAL FINANCIAL PLANNING

Mortgages

There are a bewildering array of mortgages on the market. The types include variable rate, discounted, fixed, capped and flexible. Always check for penalties for early encashment. As far as the practitioner is concerned, you may want to make one or more rooms in your next home into a therapy room or a small centre. Many lenders will not countenance this, or may require an additional interest rate as this constitutes a part Commercial Loan. There are a few however, who may not do this. A Mortgage Broker or Independent Financial Advisor will be able to help here.

Health Insurance

There are four aspects to this:

1) Long Term Disability Insurance – often known as 'permanent health insurance', which provides a regular income in the event of long term disability due to illness or injury. Premiums are paid to insurance companies who guarantee to pay income to an employed or self-employed person whose disability lasts beyond a specified deferred period. Up to 60% of income can be insured in this way. Once the waiting period is

completed (typically one to three months), and provided medical evidence proves that a person cannot work, the insurance company will pay the employed or self-employed person an income as provided under the policy until such time as the individual returns to work, dies or reaches the specified termination age (usually their retirement age) in the policy. Should the disabled person return to work part time or in a lesser, lower-paid capacity, arrangements can usually be made for the benefit to be proportionately reduced but still payable until such time as full recovery and total return to work is achieved. The income is free of tax, but a claim is subject to proof of income prior to the claim, and a maximum of 60% of taxable income is the norm these days. Policies can also be taken out to provide for business expenses and the provision of a locum, in order to protect your practice whilst you are off work. Check the small print and ensure that premiums are guaranteed not to increase over the term of cover.

2) Personal Accident & Illness Insurance – this covers both temporary total and temporary partial disablement, up to 2 years benefit (rather than to retirement age). In addition, lump sums for loss of use of limbs, faculties, joints, etc are covered for lump sum compensation in the event of an accident. Premiums are generally cheaper, but cover is annually renewable, rather than permanent, and insurers can revise their terms and exclude any serious claims made from future payments. Some policies only pay out at the end of the disablement period, or at the insurers' discretion. Others are more generous in their claims handling and pay at the end of the month. If you have had a previous Health Condition, some Health Insurers will decline to insure you, or require extra

premiums. Accident & Sickness Insurers may simply just exclude the pre-existing conditions.

3) Private Medical Insurance – as the National Health Service frequently fails to provide a speedy service for non-urgent conditions, some people feel a need for private medical insurance. These cover costs of hospitalisation, operations, medicines, fees and out-patient costs etc. Insurance companies, in an effort to provide sensible and reasonably priced plans for the general public, offer policies with an 'excess', i.e. the policyholder agrees to pay the first £50 or £100 of any claim, which can significantly reduce the pre-miums which will be payable. Furthermore, some modern plans provide private medical insurance only if the waiting period for National Health treatment exceeds six weeks. There are policies available which offer cover for osteopathy, chiropractic, homoeo-pathy, acupuncture etc. but not most other types of complementary medicine. Some policies only cover Complementary Medicine upon referral by a GP or a specialist. Practitioners should shop around for the best option if they wish to take private medical insur-ance.

4) Life and Critical Illness Cover – Life cover is a way of protecing dependants or other parties, such as a Lending Source (i.e. Bank or Building Society) in the event of you dying during an insured period. If a member of a family is stricken with a life-threatening condition, not only is the ability of that person to earn their living in jeopardy but their whole lifestyle may have to be drastically altered, which may be costly. Critical Illness Insurance will pay out a tax-free lump sum in the event of you suffering a serious illness or permanently disabling condition. Statistically you may be more likely to suffer one of

these than actually dying before the age of 65. This cover can be especially relevant if you are single and have no dependants. These protection covers are rated on a variety of factors, such as age, gender and your state of health. It is worth getting an adviser to check out the best plan for you, as there are many schemes and variations available.

Where do you go for advice?

The advice and guidance that you receive has to be paid for! Advisors are regulated by Law, and are strictly controlled. They have to study and pass examinations before they can practise, as well as having years of experience behind them. The process involves taking a Financial 'Case History', taking into account your needs and goals, and attitude to risk, which is then condensed into a plan of action for you. Since the passing of the Financial Services Act 1986 the terms 'independent financial advice' and 'independent financial adviser' have far more meaning than they ever had before. Many sources of financial advice exist, e.g. banks, building societies, insurance companies, etc., who offer their own life assurance, pension and investment products to the general public. There are other advisers who, although not employed by a large institution, are nevertheless 'tied' to one and sell their products only.

Although those who represent one company are regulated under the Act and frequently offer a highly professional service, they are unable to give an investor access to the whole marketplace and, if they are unable to meet a client's requirements from their own portfolio of contracts, they are legally obliged to recommend that their client contacts an independent financial adviser.

The independent financial adviser, or IFA, is able to consider a client's personal circumstances and needs. The advice given must be suitable for that client in order to meet the client's wishes and aspirations. This is known as 'best or most suitable advice' in terms of the Financial Services Act 1986. Be wary, however, and like any other source of advice, do your best to check out the experience and credentials of this person.

Independent financial advisers are frequently remunerated by commission paid by a product provider for the introduction of business. Fees can be charged as an alternative, usually on an hourly basis. Full details of the commission payable must be disclosed at the point of sale for pension, life assurance and investment products. If the adviser needs to recommend a course of action or a product for which no commission is payable, then a fee may be charged but the basis of remuneration should be agreed beforehand between the adviser and the client.

Of course, if you are fully conversant with financial matters, it is possible to go direct to the financial institution of your choice and buy a policy direct. You can then pay in lump sums as and when you decide and, in some cases, save on commission. But you have to be well informed, confident that you are making the right choice in a large and complicated market and able to muster the lump sum on a regular annual basis. For the majority, it is easier and more reliable to take professional advice and pay in each month.

At the time of writing, the rules are to be changed in respect of what the various advisers can sell and how they can disclose what they will advise you on.

Chapters 9 and 10 have been written by David Balen of H & L Balen & Co., established 1950, who specialise in providing services to Complementary Medicine Practitioners and their Organisations and are the largest Intermediary in this respect.

11

YOUR INTENTION FOR YOUR CLIENTS

There is usually a great depth of communication between the hands of the giver and the body of the receiver in sensitive body work, and this makes the intent of the giver profoundly important... There needs to be a desire to help, to soothe, to ease.

Leon Chaitow, *Body Tonic*

Why are some therapists really good while others are merely average? I believe it is not just a matter of training, ability, and personality, but intention. To treat clients really well, it has to be our intention to make a *positive* difference to them.

The paradox is that our intention for a good outcome runs alongside a detachment from that outcome, and the lack of a fixed idea of what that will be. In other words, we want the best for our clients without imposing on them our idea of what that best should be. This also extends to ourselves, in that we should intend to be caring, able, conscientious therapists. Florence Nightingale said that hospitals should do the sick no harm. I believe that that goes for complementary therapists too.

12

LONG TERM GOALS

The best thing about the future is that it comes one day at a time.

Abraham Lincoln

Now that we've considered so many aspects of your complementary therapy practice, it is time to return to your goals. You need to keep reviewing your goals and achievements to ensure that they are still right for you. After you've been a therapist for a while, look at how your practice is developing and evaluate your achievements so far.

- Have you achieved what you set out to do?
- How could you improve things further?
- What comes next?
- Where do you see yourself in five or ten years' time?
- Will you be continuing as you are?
- Will you be writing or lecturing?
- Will you be selling associated products?
- Will you be starting your own multi-disciplinary clinic?
- Will you be teaching?
- Will you be working in the media?

If you have taken on board the advice provided in this book, you should be well on your way to developing a satisfying, productive professional practice.

ADDRESSES

Oils and equipment

Fleur Aromatherapy   *carrier oils and essential oils*
Langston Priory Mews
Kingham
OXFORDSHIRE OX7 6UP
01608 659909

NHR   *organic oils*
5 College Terrace
Brighton
E. SUSSEX BN2 0EE
Phone: 0845 310 8066
Fax: 0870 135 2711
www.nhr.kz

Weleda UK   *homeopathic remedies and some oils*
Heanor Road
Ilkeston
DERBYSHIRE DE7 8BR
0115 944 8200
www.weleda.co.uk

Ainsworth's Pharmacy   *homeopathic supplies*
36 New Cavendish Street
London W1G 8UF
020 7935 5330
www.ainsworths.com

Plinth 2000 Ltd   *hydraulic and electric couches*
Wetheringsett Manor
Wetheringsett
Stowmarket
SUFFOLK IP14 5PP
01449 767887
www.plinth2000.com

Darley Therapy Equipment   *couches*
5 Restormel Estate
Lostwithiel
CORNWALL PL22 0HG
01208 873200
www.darley-couches.co.uk

Marshcouch   *couches, covers, accessories*
36 Glebe Close
Hemel Hempstead
HERTFORDSHIRE HP3 9PA
01442 263199

New Concept   *bodywork and therapy equipment*
2 Bermuda Road
Ransomes Euro Park
Ipswich
SUFFOLK IP3 9RU
01473 720572
email: info@new-concept.co.uk

Osteopathic Supplies Limited   *complementary and*
70 Belmont Road   *physical healthcare*
Hereford
HEREFORDSHIRE HR2 7JW
01432 263969
email: sales@o-s-l.com
www.o-s-l.com

Clothing

DK Profashion
1 Bank Street
Tonbridge
KENT TN9 1BL
01732 359789

Alison Bell Fabric Designs
Gravel Pit Cottages
High Toynton
Horncastle
LINCOLNSHIRE LN9 6NN
01507 526591
email: alisonbell@tjs.co.uk
www.yoga-clothing.co.uk

Insurance

H & L Balen and Company   *specialist insurance*
33 Graham Road   *brokers and independent*
Great Malvern   *financial advisers*
WORCESTERSHIRE WR14 2HU
01684 893006

Ecology Insurance Brokers Ltd
Oaklands
Postmans Lane
Little Baddow
Chelmsford
ESSEX CM3 4SF
01245 225198
email: admin@ecologyinsurance.co.uk

Umbrella Organisations

British Massage Therapy Council
01865 774123
www.bmtc.co.uk

British Complementary Medicine Association
PO Box 2074
Seaford
EAST SUSSEX BN25 1HQ
0845 345 5977
www.bcma.co.uk

British Federation of Massage Practitioners
78 Meadow Street
Preston
LANCASHIRE PR1 1TS
01772 881063
www.jolanta.co.uk

Aromatherapy Organisations Council
PO Box 19834
London SE25 6WF
020 8251 7912

Guild of Complementary Practitioners
Liddell House
Liddell Close
Finchampstead
BERKSHIRE RG40 4NS
0118 973 5757
www.gcpnet.com

Institute for Complementary Medicine
PO Box 194
London SE16 1QZ
020 7237 5165
www.icmedicine.co.uk

Workshops and lectures

Celia Johnson can be contacted at
www.successfultherapist.co.uk
Email: Celia@successfultherapist.co.uk

The Data Protection Act

Wycliffe House
Water Lane
Wilmslow
CHESHIRE SK9 5AF
01625 545700
www.dataprotection.gov.uk

Further reading

Judy Hall, *The Art of Psychic Protection* (Findhorn Press)
Stuart Wilde, *The Trick to Money is Having Some* (Hay
    House publishing)
Lorna Galbraith-Ryan and Lois Graessle, *Money's no
    Object* (Mandarin Books)
Val Falloon, *How to get more clients* (Brainwave)
Richard Reoch, *Dying Well* (Gaia Books)
Patricia McNamara, *Massage for People with Cancer*
    (Wandsworth Cancer Support Centre, 020 7924 3924)

Book Clubs

Cygnus Book Club
PO Box 15
Llandeilo
CARMARTHENSHIRE SA19 6YX
01550 777701
www.cygnus-books.co.uk

The Tao of Books
Station Warehouse
Station Road
Pulham Market
SUFFOLK IP21 4XF
01379 676000
www.taobook.com

Mind, Body and Spirit
Birmingham B26 3UE
www.join.mind-body-spirit.co.uk

Journals

Journal of Alternative and Complementary Medicine,
available on subscription
Green Library
9 Rickett Street
London SW6 1RU
020 7385 0012

What Doctors Don't Tell You, available on subscription
Satellite House
2 Salisbury Road
London SW19 4EZ
020 8944 9555
www.wddty.co.uk

Positive Health, available from newsagents and on
subscription
1 Queen Square
Bristol BS1 4JQ
www.positivehealth.com
0117 983 8851

Here's Health, available from newsagents and on
subscription
Tower Publishing Services
Tower House
Sovereign Park
Lathkill Street
Market Harborough
LEICESTERSHIRE LE16 9EF
01858 438869 (for subscriptions)
www.ukmagazines.co.uk

INDEX